Dash Diet Cooking Guide for Beginners

The Perfect Cookbook for a Fit and Healthy Lifestyle

Eleonore Barlow

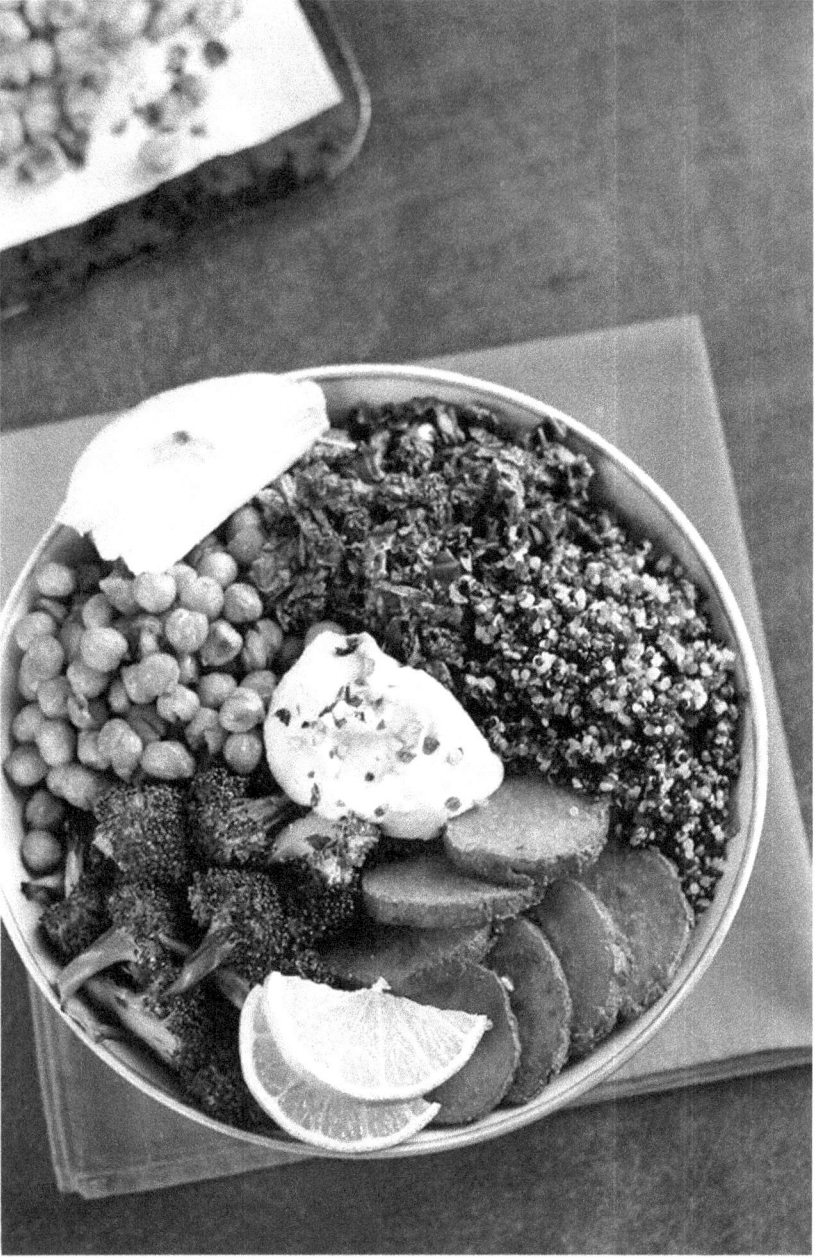

Table of Contents

AMAZING AND HEALTHY GRANOLA BOWL 6

CINNAMON AND PUMPKIN PORRIDGE MEDLEY 8

QUINOA AND DATE BOWL 10

CRISPY TOFU 12

HEARTY PUMPKIN OATS 15

WHOLESOME PUMPKIN PIE OATMEAL 17

POWER-PACKED OATMEAL 19

SAUCY GARLIC GREENS..21

GARDEN SALAD 23

SPICY CABBAGE DISH.. 26

EXTREME BALSAMIC CHICKEN 28

ENJOYABLE SPINACH AND BEAN MEDLEY 30

BROWN BUTTER DUCK BREAST 32

GENEROUS GARLIC BREAD STICK.. 34

CAULIFLOWER BREAD STICK 36

BACON AND CHICKEN GARLIC WRAP 39

PORTUGUESE KALE AND SAUSAGE SOUP 41

DAZZLING PIZZA SOUP 43

MESMERIZING LENTIL SOUP 45

ORGANICALLY HEALTHY CHICKEN SOUP 48

POTATO AND ASPARAGUS BISQUE 50

CABBAGE AND LEEK SOUP.. 52

ONION SOUP... 54

CARROT, GINGER AND TURMERIC SOUP 56

OFFBEAT SQUASH SOUP 58

SIMPLE ONE POT MUSSELS... 60

LEMON PEPPER AND SALMON 62

SIMPLE SAUTÉED GARLIC AND PARSLEY SCALLOPS 65

SALMON AND CUCUMBER PLATTER 67

TUNA PATÉ 69

BEEF WITH PEA PODS 70

WHOLE-GRAIN ROTINI WITH GROUND PORK 73

ROASTED PORK LOIN WITH HERBS 75

GARLIC LIME PORK CHOPS 77

THE MOST ELEGANT PARSLEY SOUFFLÉ EVER 79

FENNEL AND ALMOND BITES 80

FEISTY COCONUT FUDGE 81

NO BAKE CHEESECAKE 83

EASY CHIA SEED PUMPKIN PUDDING 85

LOVELY BLUEBERRY PUDDING 86

DECISIVE LIME AND STRAWBERRY POPSICLE 87

AUTHENTIC GINGER AND BERRY SMOOTHIE 88

A GLASSFUL OF KALE AND SPINACH 90

GREEN TEA, TURMERIC, AND MANGO SMOOTHIE 92

THE GREAT ANTI-OXIDANT GLASS 94

FRESH MINTY SMOOTHIE 96

APPLE SLICES 98

ELEGANT CASHEW SAUCE 100

LOVELY JAPANESE CABBAGE DISH 102

ALMOND BUTTERY GREEN CABBAGE 104

Amazing and Healthy Granola Bowl

Serving: 6

Prep Time: 5 minutes

Cook Time: 25 minutes

Ingredients:

1-ounce Porridge oats

2 teaspoons maple syrup

Cooking spray as needed

4 medium bananas

4 pots of Caramel

Layered Fromage Frais

5-ounce fresh fruit salad, such as strawberries, blueberries, and raspberries

¼ ounce pumpkin seeds

¼ ounce sunflower seeds

¼ ounce dry chia seeds

¼ ounce desiccated coconut

How To:

1. Preheat your oven to 300 degrees F.

2. Take a baking tray and line with baking paper.

3. Take an outsized bowl and add oats, syrup, and seeds.

4. Spread mix on a baking tray.

5. Spray copra oil on top and bake for 20 minutes, ensuring to stay stirring from time to time.

6. Sprinkle coconut after the primary quarter-hour.

7. Remove from oven and let it cool.

8. Take a bowl and layer sliced bananas on top of the Fromage Fraise.

9. Spread the cooled granola mix on top and serve with a topping of berries.

10. Enjoy!

Nutrition (Per Serving)

Calories: 446

Fat: 29g

Carbohydrates: 37g

Protein: 13g

Cinnamon and Pumpkin Porridge Medley

Serving: 2

Prep Time: 10 minutes

Cook Time: 15 minutes

Ingredients:

1 cup unsweetened almond/coconut milk

1 cup of water

1 cup uncooked quinoa

½ cup pumpkin puree

1 teaspoon ground cinnamon

2 tablespoons ground flaxseed meal

Juice of 1 lemon

How To:

1.	Take a pot and place it over medium-high heat.

2.	Whisk in water, almond milk and convey the combination to a boil.

3.	Stir in quinoa, cinnamon, and pumpkin.

4.	Reduce heat to low and simmer for 10 minutes until the liquid has evaporated.

5.	Remove from the warmth and stir in flaxseed meal.

6.	Transfer porridge to small bowls.

7.	Sprinkle juice and add pumpkin seeds on top.

8.	Serve and enjoy!

Nutrition (Per Serving)

Calories: 245

Fat: 1g

Carbohydrates: 59g

Protein: 4g

Quinoa and Date Bowl

Serving: 2

Prep Time: 10 minutes

Cook Time: 15 minutes

Ingredients:

1 date, pitted and chopped finely

½ cup red quinoa, dried

1 cup unsweetened almond milk

1/8 teaspoon vanilla extract

¼ cup fresh strawberries, hulled and sliced 1/8 teaspoon ground cinnamon

How To:

1.   Take a pan and place it over low heat.

2.   Add quinoa, almond milk, cinnamon, vanilla, and cook for about quarter-hour, ensuring to stay stirring from time to time.

3. Garnish with strawberries and enjoy!

Nutrition (Per Serving)

Calories: 195

Fat: 4.4g

Carbohydrates: 32g

Protein: 7g

Crispy Tofu

Serving: 8

Prep Time: 5 minutes

Cook Time: 20-30 minutes

Ingredients:

1-pound extra-firm tofu, drained and sliced

2 tablespoons olive oil

1 cup almond meal

1 tablespoons yeast

½ teaspoon onion powder ½ teaspoon garlic powder ½ teaspoon oregano

How To:

1.   Add all ingredients except tofu and vegetable oil during a shallow bowl.

2.   Mix well.

3.   Preheat your oven to 400 degrees F.

4.   during a wide bowl, add the almond meal and blend well.

5.   Brush tofu with vegetable oil, read the combination and coat well.

6.   Line a baking sheet with parchment paper.

7.   Transfer coated tofu to the baking sheet.

8.   Bake for 20-30 minutes, ensuring to flip once until golden brown.

9.   Serve and enjoy!

Nutrition (Per Serving)

Calories: 282

Fat: 20g

Carbohydrates: 9g

Protein: 12g

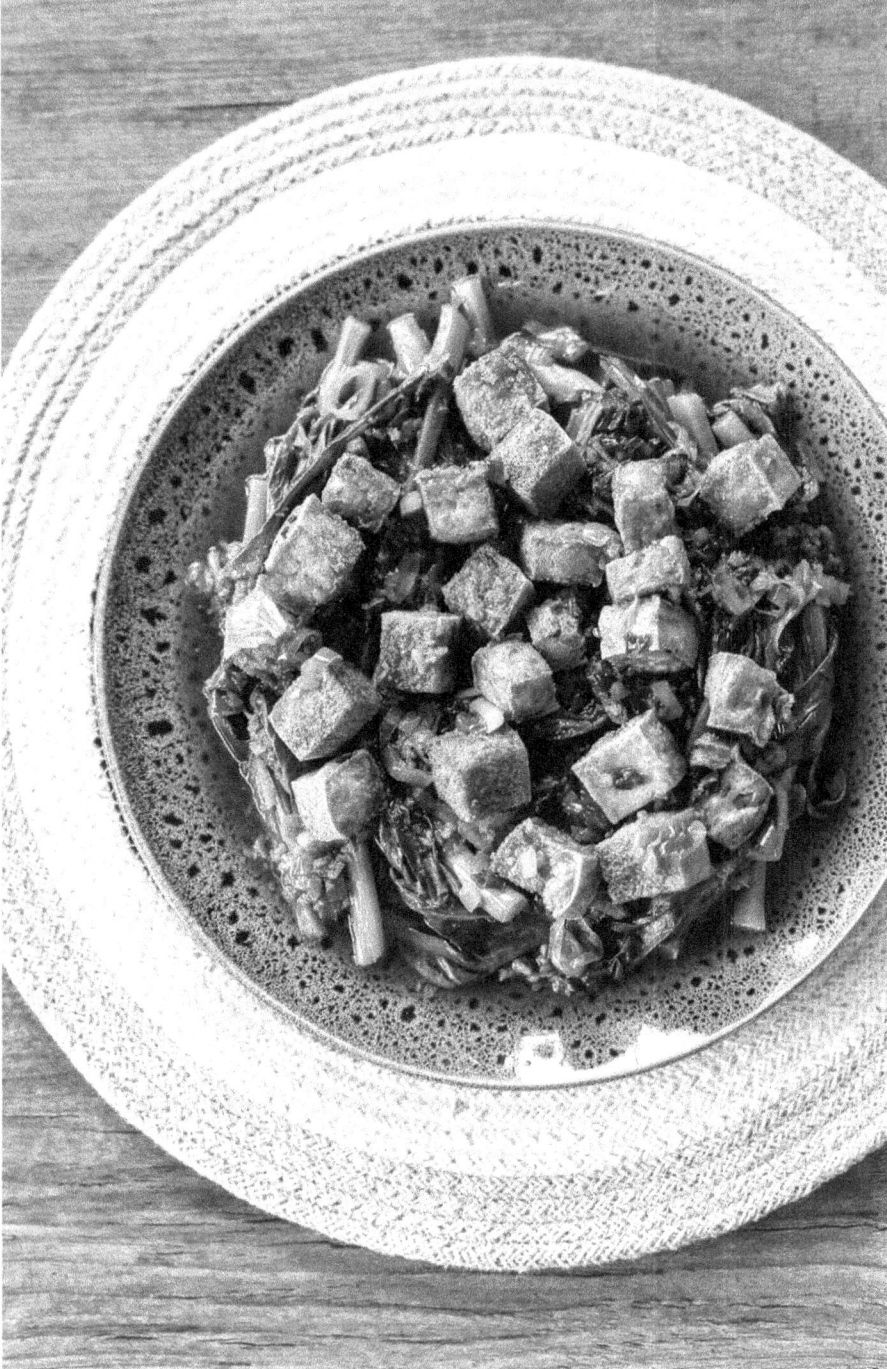

Hearty Pumpkin Oats

Serving: 3

Prep Time: 5 minutes

Cook Time: 8 minutes

Ingredients:

1 cup quick-cooking rolled oats

¾ cup almond milk

½ cup canned pumpkin puree

¼ teaspoon pumpkin pie spice

1 teaspoon ground cinnamon

How To:

1.   Take a secure microwave bowl and add oats, almond milk, and microwave on high for 1-2 minutes.

2.   Add more almond milk if needed to realize your required consistency.

3.   Cook for 30 seconds more.

4.   Stir in pumpkin puree, pie spice, ground cinnamon.

5.   Heat gently and enjoy!

Nutrition (Per Serving)

Calories: 229

Fat: 4g

Carbohydrates: 38g

Protein:10g

Wholesome Pumpkin Pie Oatmeal

Serving: 2

Prep Time: 10 minutes

Cook Time: 10 minutes

Smart Points: 6

Ingredients:

½ cup canned pumpkin, low sodium

Mashed banana as needed

¾ cup unsweetened almond milk

½ teaspoon pumpkin pie spice

1 cup oats

How To:

1.   Mash banana employing a fork and blend within the remaining ingredients (except oats) and blend well.

2.   Add oats and finely stir.

3.   Transfer mixture to a pot and let the oats cook until it's absorbed the liquid and is tender.

4.   Serve and enjoy!

Nutrition (Per Serving)

Calories: 264

Fat: 4g

Carbohydrates: 52g

Protein: 7g

Power-Packed Oatmeal

Serving: 2

Prep Time: 10-15 minutes

Cook Time: 5 minutes

Ingredients:

¼ cup quick-cooking oats

¼ cup almond milk

2 tablespoons low fat Greek yogurt

¼ banana, mashed

2-1/4 tablespoons flaxseed meal

How To:

1.   Whisk altogether of the ingredients during a bowl.

2.   Transfer the bowl to your fridge and let it refrigerate for quarter-hour.

3.   Serve and enjoy!

Nutrition (Per Serving)

Calories:

Fat: 11g

Carbohydrates: 27g

Protein: 10g

Saucy Garlic Greens

Serving: 4

Prep Time: 5 minutes

Cook Time: 20 minutes

Ingredients:

1 bunch of leafy greens Sauce

½ cup cashews soaked in water for 10 minutes ¼ cup water

1 tablespoon lemon juice

1 teaspoon coconut aminos

1 clove peeled whole clove

1/8 teaspoon of flavored vinegar

How To:

1.   Make the sauce by draining and discarding the soaking water from your cashews and add the cashews to a blender.

2.   Add water, juice, flavored vinegar, coconut aminos, garlic.

3.   Blitz until you've got a smooth cream and transfer to bowl.

4.   Add ½ cup of water to the pot.

5.   Place the steamer basket to the pot and add the greens within the basket.

6.   Lock the lid and steam for 1 minute.

7.   Quick-release the pressure.

8.   Transfer the steamed greens to strainer and extract excess water.

9.   Place the greens into a bowl.

10.   Add lemon aioli and toss.

11.   Enjoy!

Nutrition (Per Serving)

Calories: 77

Fat: 5g

Carbohydrates: 0g

Protein: 2g

Garden Salad

Serving: 6

Prep Time: 5 minutes

Cook Time: 20 minutes

Ingredients:

1-pound raw peanuts in shell

1 bay leaf

2 medium-sized chopped up tomatoes

½ cup diced up green pepper

½ cup diced up sweet onion

¼ cup finely diced hot pepper

¼ cup diced up celery

2 tablespoons olive oil

¾ teaspoon flavored vinegar

¼ teaspoon freshly ground black pepper

How To:

1. Boil your peanuts for 1 minute and rinse them.

2. The skins are going to be soft, so discard the skin.

3. Add 2 cups of water to the moment Pot.

4. Add herb and peanuts.

5. Lock the lid and cook on high for 20 minutes.

6. Drain the water.

7. Take an outsized bowl and add the peanuts, diced up vegetables.

8. Whisk in vegetable oil, juice, pepper in another bowl.

9. Pour the mixture over the salad and blend.

10. Enjoy!

Nutrition (Per Serving)

Calories: 140

Fat: 4g

Carbohydrates: 24g

Protein: 5g

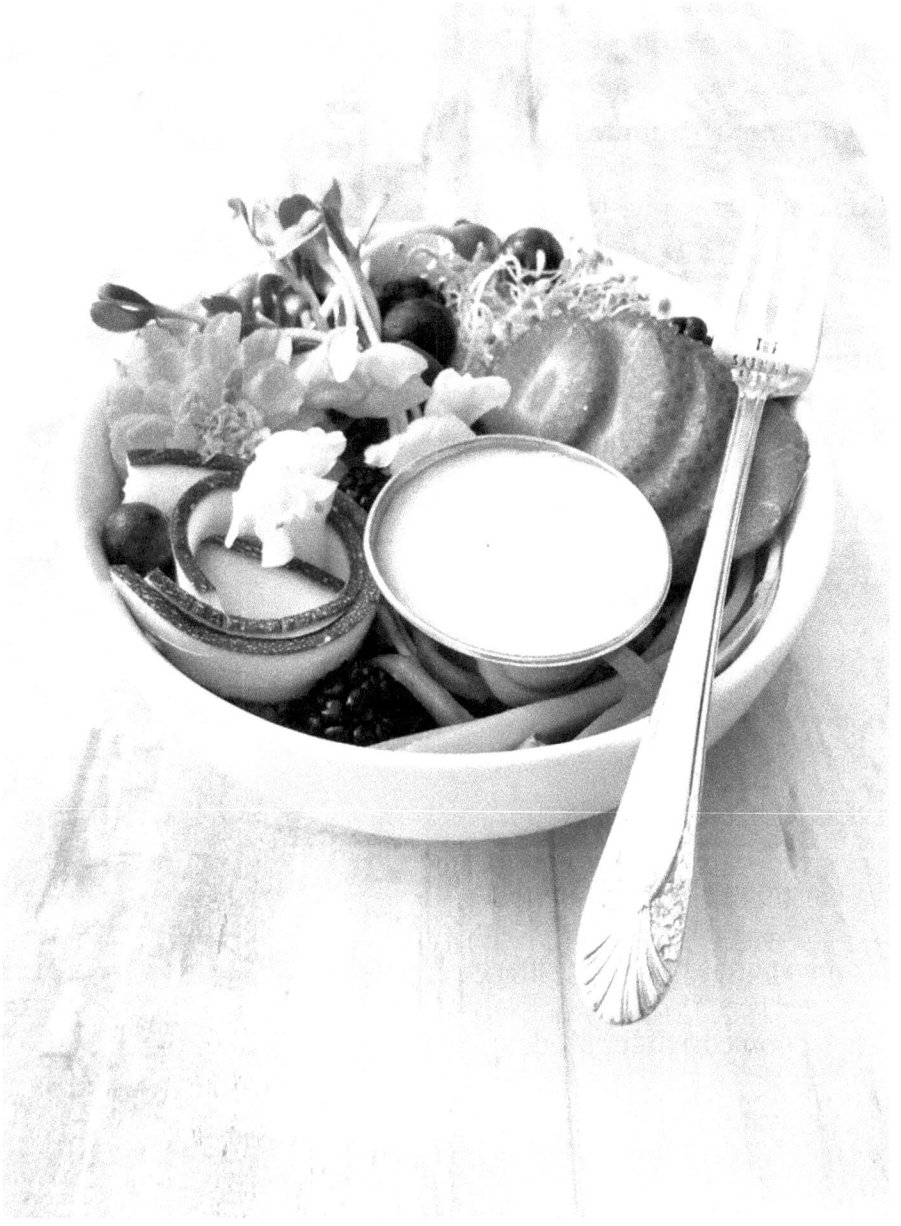

Spicy Cabbage Dish

Serving: 4

Prep Time: 10 minutes

Cooking Time: 4 hours

Ingredients:

2 yellow onions, chopped

10 cups red cabbage, shredded

1 cup plums, pitted and chopped

1 teaspoon cinnamon powder

1 garlic clove, minced

1 teaspoon cumin seeds

¼ teaspoon cloves, ground

2 tablespoons red wine vinegar

1 teaspoon coriander seeds

½ cup water

How To:

1.   Add cabbage, onion, plums, garlic, cumin, cinnamon, cloves, vinegar, coriander and water to your Slow Cooker.

2.   Stir well.

3.   Place lid and cook on LOW for 4 hours.

4.   Divide between serving platters.

5.   Enjoy!

Nutrition (Per Serving)

Calories: 197

Fat: 1g

Carbohydrates: 14g

Protein: 3g

Extreme Balsamic Chicken

Serving: 4

Prep Time: 10 minutes

Cook Time: 35 minutes

Ingredients:

3 boneless chicken breasts, skinless

Sunflower seeds to taste

¼ cup almond flour

2/3 cups low-fat chicken broth

1 ½ teaspoons arrowroot

½ cup low sugar raspberry preserve

1 ½ tablespoons balsamic vinegar

How To:

1.   Cut pigeon breast into bite-sized pieces and season them with seeds.

2.   Dredge the chicken pieces in flour and shake off any excess.

3.   Take a non-stick skillet and place it over medium heat.

4.   Add chicken to the skillet and cook for quarter-hour , ensuring to show them half-way through.

5.   Remove chicken and transfer to platter.

6.   Add arrowroot, broth, raspberry preserve to the skillet and stir.

7.   Stir in balsamic vinegar and reduce heat to low, stir-cook for a couple of minutes.

8.   Transfer the chicken back to the sauce and cook for quarter-hour more.

9.   Serve and enjoy!

Nutrition (Per Serving)

Calories: 546

Fat: 35g

Carbohydrates: 11g

Protein: 44g

Enjoyable Spinach and Bean Medley

Serving: 4

Prep Time: 10 minutes

Cooking Time: 4 hours

Ingredients:

5 carrots, sliced

1 ½ cups great northern beans, dried

2 garlic cloves, minced

1 yellow onion, chopped

Pepper to taste

½ teaspoon oregano, dried

5 ounces baby spinach

4 ½ cups low sodium veggie stock

2 teaspoons lemon peel, grated

3 tablespoon lemon juice

How To:

1.   Add beans, onion, carrots, garlic, oregano and stock to your Slow Cooker.

2.   Stir well.

3.   Place lid and cook on HIGH for 4 hours.

4.   Add spinach, juice and lemon rind.

5.   Stir and let it sit for five minutes.

6.   Divide between serving platters and enjoy!

Nutrition (Per Serving)

Calories: 219

Fat: 8g

Carbohydrates: 14g

Protein: 8g

Brown Butter Duck Breast

Serving: 3

Prep Time: 5 minutes

Cook Time: 25 minutes

Ingredients:

1 whole 6-ounce duck breast, skin on

Pepper to taste

1 head radicchio, 4 ounces, core removed ¼ cup unsalted butter

6 fresh sage leaves, sliced

How To:

1.   Pre-heat your oven to 400-degree F.

2.   Pat duck breast dry with towel.

3.   Season with pepper.

4.   Place duck breast in skillet and place it over medium heat, sear for 3-4 minutes all sides

5.   Turn breast over and transfer skillet to oven.

6.   Roast for 10 minutes (uncovered).

7.   Cut radicchio in half.

8.   Remove and discard the woody white core and thinly slice the leaves.

9.   Keep them on the side.

10.   Remove skillet from oven.

11.   Transfer duck breast, fat side up to chopping board and let it rest.

12.   Re-heat your skillet over medium heat.

13. Add unsalted butter, sage and cook for 3-4 minutes.

14.   Cut duck into 6 equal slices.

15.   Divide radicchio between 2 plates, top with slices of duck breast and drizzle browned butter and sage.

16.   Enjoy!

Nutrition (Per Serving)

Calories: 393

Fat: 33g

Carbohydrates: 2g

Protein: 22g

Generous Garlic Bread Stick

Serving: 8 breadsticks

Prep Time: 15 minutes

Cooking Time: 15 minutes

Ingredients:

¼ cup almond butter, softened

1 teaspoon garlic powder

2 cups almond flour

½ tablespoon baking powder

1 tablespoon Psyllium husk powder

¼ teaspoon sunflower seeds

3 tablespoons almond butter, melted

1 egg

¼ cup boiling water

How To:

1.   Pre-heat your oven to 400 degrees F.

2. Line baking sheet with parchment paper and keep it on the side.

3. Beat almond butter with garlic powder and keep it on the side.

4. Add almond flour, leaven, husk, sunflower seeds during a bowl and blend in almond butter and egg, mix well.

5. Pour boiling water within the mix and stir until you've got a pleasant dough.

6. Divide the dough into 8 balls and roll into breadsticks.

7. Place on baking sheet and bake for quarter-hour.

8. Brush each persist with garlic almond butter and bake for five minutes more.

9. Serve and enjoy!

Nutrition (Per Serving)

Total Carbs: 7g

Fiber: 2g

Protein: 7g

Fat: 24g

Cauliflower Bread Stick

Serving: 5 breadsticks

Prep Time: 10 minutes

Cooking Time: 48 minutes

Ingredients:

1 cup cashew cheese/ kite ricotta cheese

1 tablespoon organic almond butter

1 whole egg

½ teaspoon Italian seasoning

¼ teaspoon red pepper flakes

1/8 teaspoon kosher sunflower seeds

2 cups cauliflower rice, cooked for 3 minutes in microwave

3 teaspoons garlic, minced

Parmesan cheese, grated

How To:

1.   Pre-heat your oven to 350 degrees F.

2.   Add almond butter during a small pan and melt over low heat

3.   Add red pepper flakes, garlic to the almond butter and cook for 2-3 minutes.

4.   Add garlic and almond butter mix to the bowl with cooked cauliflower and add the Italian seasoning.

5.   Season with sunflower seeds and blend, refrigerate for 10 minutes.

6.   Add cheese and eggs to the bowl and blend.

7.   Place a layer of parchment paper at rock bottom of a 9 x 9 baking dish and grease with cooking spray, add egg and mozzarella cheese mix to the cauliflower mix.

8.   Add mix to the pan and smooth to a skinny layer with the palms of your hand.

9.   Bake for half-hour , remove from oven and top with few shakes of parmesan and mozzarella.

10.   Cook for 8 minutes more.

11.   Enjoy!

Nutrition (Per Serving)

Total Carbs: 11.5g

Fiber: 2g

Protein: 10.7g

Fat: 20g

Bacon and Chicken Garlic Wrap

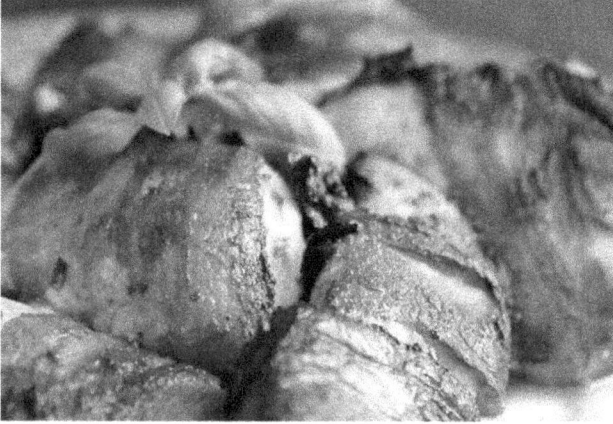

Serving: 4

Prep Time: 15 minutes

Cook Time: 10 minutes

Ingredients:

1 chicken fillet, cut into small cubes

8-9 thin slices bacon, cut to fit cubes

6 garlic cloves, minced

How To:

1.   Pre-heat your oven to 400 degrees F.

2.   Line a baking tray with aluminum foil .

3.   Add minced garlic to a bowl and rub each chicken piece with it.

4.   Wrap a bacon piece around each garlic chicken bite.

5.   Secure with toothpick.

6.   Transfer bites to baking sheet, keeping a touch little bit of space between them.

7.   Bake for about 15-20 minutes until crispy.

8.   Serve and enjoy!

Nutrition (Per Serving)

Calories: 260

Fat: 19g

Carbohydrates: 5g

Protein: 22g

Portuguese Kale and Sausage Soup

Serving: 4

Prep Time: 10 minutes

Cook Time: 35 minutes

Ingredients:

1 yellow onion, chopped

16 ounces sausage, chopped

3 sweet potatoes, chopped

4cups chicken stock1 pound kale, chopped pepper as needed

How To:

1.   Take a pot and place it over medium heat.

2.   Add sausage and brown each side.

3.   Transfer to bowl.

4.   Heat pot again over medium heat.

5.   Add onion and stir for five minutes.

6.   Add stock, sweet potatoes, stir and convey to a simmer.

7. Cook for 20 minutes.

8. Use an immersion blender to blend.

9. Add kale and pepper and simmer for two minutes over low heat.

10. Ladle soup to bowls and top with sausage with pieces.

11. Serve and enjoy!

Nutrition (Per Serving)

Calories: 200

Fat: 2g

Carbohydrates: 6g

Protein:8g

Dazzling Pizza Soup

Serving: 6

Prep Time: 5 minutes

Cook Time: 30 minutes

Ingredients:

12 ounces chicken meat, sliced

4 ounces uncured pepperoni

1 can 25 ounces marinara

1 can 14.5 ounces fire roasted tomatoes

1 large onion, diced

15 ounces mushrooms, sliced

1 can 3 ounce sliced black olives

tablespoon dried oregano

1 teaspoon garlic powder

½ teaspoon salt

How To:

1.   Take large sized saucepan and add within the peperoni, chicken meat, marinara, onions, tomatoes, mushroom, oregano, olives, salt and garlic powder.

2.   Cook the mixture for half-hour over medium level heat and soften the mushroom and onions.

3.   Serve hot.

Nutrition (Per Serving)

Calories: 90

Fat: 2g

Carbohydrates: 17g

Protein: 3g

Mesmerizing Lentil Soup

Serving: 4

Prep Time: 10 minutes

Cooking Time: 8 hours

Ingredients:

1 pound dried lentils, soaked overnight and rinsed carrots, peeled and chopped

1 celery stalk, chopped

1 onion, chopped

6 cups vegetables broth

1 ½ teaspoons garlic powder

1 teaspoon ground cumin

1 teaspoon smoked paprika

1 teaspoon dried thyme

¼ teaspoon liquid smoke

¼ teaspoon salt

¼ teaspoon ground pepper

How To:

1.   Add listed ingredients to Slow Cooker and stir well.

2.   Place lid and cook for 8 hours on LOW.

3.   Stir and serve.

4.   Enjoy!

Nutrition (Per Serving)

Calories: 307

Fat: 1g

Carbohydrates: 56g

Protein: 20g

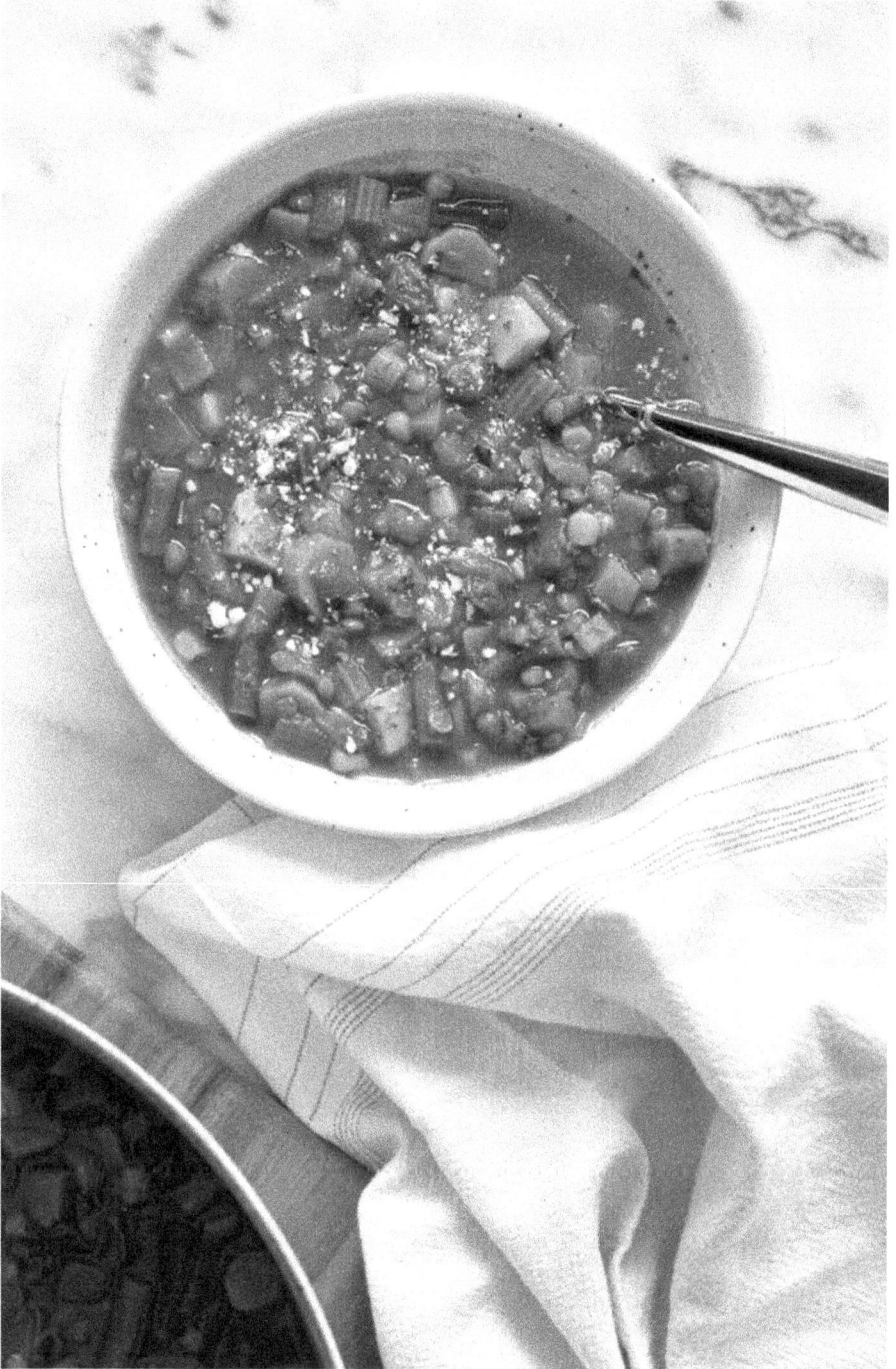

Organically Healthy Chicken Soup

Serving: 4

Prep Time: 10 minutes

Cook Time: 12-15 minutes

Ingredients:

cans (14 ounces each) low sodium chicken broth 2 cups water

1 cup twisted spaghetti

¼ teaspoon pepper

cups mixed vegetables (such as broccoli, carrots etc.)

1 and ½ cups chicken, cooked and cubed

1 tablespoon fresh basil, snipped

¼ cup parmesan, finely shredded

How To:

1.   Take a Dutch Oven and add broth, water, pepper and bring the mixture to a boil. 2. Gently stir in pasta and wait until the mixture reaches boiling point again,

2.   Lower down the heat and let the mixture simmer for 5 minutes (covered).

3.   Remove lid and stir in the vegetables, return the mixture boil and lower down heat once again.

4.   Cover and let it simmer over low heat for 5-8 minutes until the pasta and veggies and tender and cooked.

5.   Stir in cooked chicken and garnish with basil.

6.   Serve with a topping of parmesan.

7.   Enjoy!

Nutrition Values (Per Serving)

Calories: 400

Fat: 9g

Carbohydrates: 37g

Protein: 45g

Potato and Asparagus Bisque

Serving: 4

Prep Time: 5 minutes

Cook Time: 6 minutes

Ingredients:

1 ½ pound asparagus

2 pounds sweet potatoes

cups vegetable broth

1 large sized onion

8 cloves garlic

2 tablespoons dried dill

2 tablespoons flavored vinegar

3-4 cups almond milk

4 tablespoons Dijon mustard

4 tablespoons yeast

How To:

1.   Add the listed ingredients (except milk, mustard and yeast) to your pot.

2.   Lock the lid and cook on HIGH pressure for 6 minutes.

3.   Release the pressure naturally.

4.   Open the lid and add almond milk, yeast and mustard.

5.   Puree using immersion blender.

6.   Serve over rice.

7.   Enjoy!

Nutrition (Per Serving)

Calories: 430

Fat: 12g

Carbohydrates: 77g

Protein: 6g

Cabbage and Leek Soup

Serving: 4

Prep Time: 10 minutes

Cook Time: 25 minutes

Ingredients:

2 tablespoons coconut oil

½ head chopped up cabbage

3-4 diced ribs celery

2-3 carefully cleaned and chopped leeks

1 diced bell pepper

2-3 diced carrots

2/3 cloves minced garlic

4 cups chicken broth

1 teaspoon Italian seasoning

1 teaspoon Creole seasoning

Black pepper as needed

2-3 cups mixed salad greens

How To:

1. Set your pot to Sauté mode and add coconut oil.

2. Allow the oil to heat up.

3. Add the veggies (except salad greens) starting from the carrot, making sure to stir well after each vegetable addition.

4. Make sure to add the garlic last.

5. Season with Italian seasoning, black pepper and Creole seasoning.

6. Add broth and lock the lid.

7. Cook on SOUP mode for 20 minutes.

8. Release the pressure naturally and add salad greens, stir well and allow to sit for a while.

9. Allow for a few minutes to wilt the veggies.

10. Season with a bit of flavored vinegar and pepper and enjoy!

Nutrition (Per Serving)

Calories: 32

Fat: 0g

Carbohydrates: 4g

Protein: 2g

Onion Soup

Serving: 4

Prep Time: 10 minutes

Cook Time: 3 hours

Ingredients:

2 tablespoons avocado oil

yellow onions, cut into halved and sliced Black pepper to taste 5 cups beef stock

3 thyme sprigs

1 tablespoon tomato paste

How To:

1.   Take a pot and place it over medium high heat.

2.   Add onion and thyme and stir.

3.   Reduce heat to low and cook for 30 minutes.

4.   Uncover pot and cook onions for 1 hour and 30 minutes more, stirring often.

5.   Add tomato paste, stock and stir.

6.   Simmer for 1 hour more.

7.   Ladle soup into bowls and enjoy!

Nutrition (Per Serving)

Calories: 200

Fat: 4g

Carbohydrates: 6g

Protein: 8g

Carrot, Ginger and Turmeric Soup

Serving: 4

Prep Time: 15 minutes

Cook Time: 40 minutes

Ingredients:

cups chicken broth

¼ cup full fat coconut milk, unsweetened ¾ pound carrots, peeled and chopped 1 teaspoon turmeric, ground

2 teaspoons ginger, grated

1 yellow onion, chopped

2 garlic cloves, peeled

Pinch of pepper

How To:

1.   Take a stockpot and add all the ingredients except coconut milk into it.

2.   Place stockpot over medium heat.

3.   Bring to a boil.

4.   Reduce heat to simmer for 40 minutes.

5.   Remove the bay leaf.

6.   Blend the soup until smooth by using an immersion blender.

7.   Add the coconut milk and stir.

8.   Serve immediately and enjoy!

Nutrition (Per Serving)

Calories: 79

Fat: 4g

Carbohydrates: 7g

Protein: 4g

Offbeat Squash Soup

Serving: 4

Prep Time: 10 minutes

Cook Time: 50 minutes

Ingredients:

1 butternut squash, cut in halve lengthwise and deseeded

14 ounces coconut milk

Pinch of salt

Black pepper to taste

Handful of parsley, chopped

Pinch of nutmeg, ground

How To:

1.   Add butternut squash halves on a lined baking sheet.

2.   Place in oven and bake for 45 minutes at 350 degrees F.

3.   Leave squash to cool down and scoop out the flesh to a pot.

4. Add half of the coconut milk to the pot and blend using immersion blender.

5. Heat soup over medium-low heat and add remaining coconut milk.

6. Add a pinch of salt, black pepper to taste.

7. Add nutmeg, parsley and blend using an immersion blender once again for a few seconds.

8. Cook for 4 minutes.

9. Serve and enjoy!

Nutrition (Per Serving)

Calories: 144

Fat: 10g

Carbohydrates: 7g

Protein: 2g

Simple One Pot Mussels

Serving: 4

Prep Time: 10 minutes

Cook Time: 5 minutes

Ingredients:

2 tablespoons butter

2 chopped shallots

minced garlic cloves

½ cup broth

½ cup white wine

2 pounds cleaned mussels

Lemon and parsley for serving

How To:

1.   Clean the mussels and take away the beard.

2.   Discard any mussels that don't close when tapped against a tough surface.

3.   Set your pot to Sauté mode and add chopped onion and butter.

4.   Stir and sauté onions.

5.   Add garlic and cook for 1 minute.

6.   Add broth and wine.

7.   Lock the lid and cook for five minutes on high.

8.   Release the pressure naturally over 10 minutes.

9.   Serve with a sprinkle of parsley and enjoy!

Nutrition (Per Serving)

Calories: 286

Fats: 14g

Carbs: 12g

Protein: 28g

Lemon Pepper and Salmon

Serving: 3

Prep Time: 5 minutes

Cook Time: 6 minutes

Ingredients:

¾ cup water

Few sprigs of parsley, basil, tarragon, basil 1 pound of salmon, skin on

teaspoons ghee

¼ teaspoon salt

½ teaspoon pepper

½ lemon, thinly sliced

1 whole carrot, julienned

How To:

1.   Set your pot to Sauté mode and water and herbs.

2.   Place a steamer rack inside your pot and place salmon.

3. Drizzle the ghee on top of the salmon and season with salt and pepper.

4. Cover lemon slices.

5. Lock the lid and cook on high for 3 minutes.

6. Release the pressure naturally over 10 minutes.

7. Transfer the salmon to a serving platter.

8. Set your pot to Sauté mode and add vegetables.

9. Cook for 1-2 minutes.

10. Serve with vegetables and salmon.

11. Enjoy!

Nutrition (Per Serving)

Calories: 464

Fat: 34g

Carbohydrates: 3g

Protein: 34g

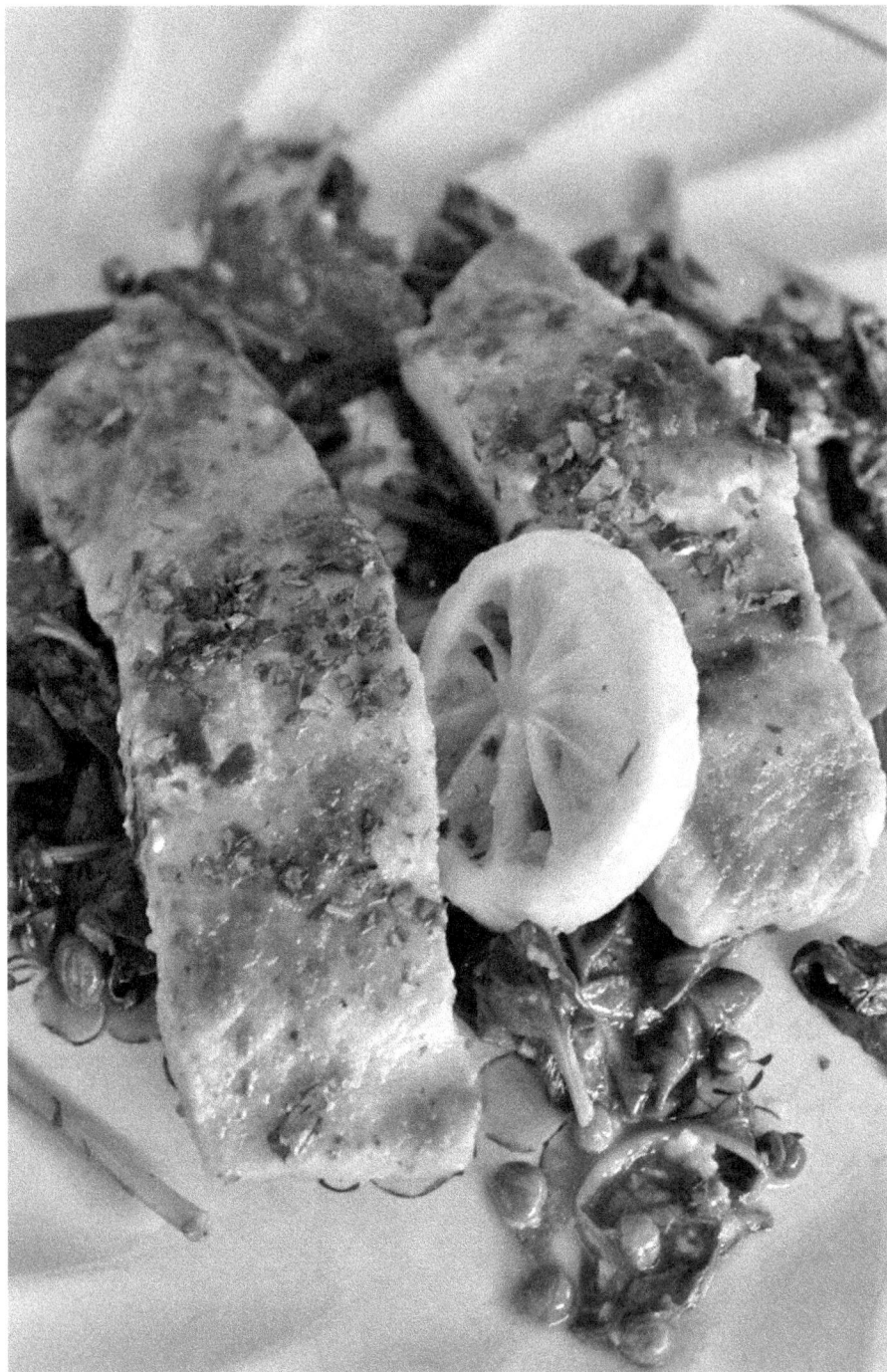

Simple Sautéed Garlic and Parsley Scallops

Serving: 4

Prep Time: 5 minutes

Cook Time: 25 minutes

Ingredients:

8 tablespoons almond butter

2 garlic cloves, minced

16 large sea scallops

Sunflower seeds and pepper to taste

1 ½ tablespoons olive oil

How To:

1.   Seasons scallops with sunflower seeds and pepper.

2.   Take a skillet, place it over medium heat, add oil and let it heat up.

3.   Sauté scallops for two minutes per side, repeat until all scallops are cooked.

4.   Add almond butter to the skillet and let it melt.

5.   Stir in garlic and cook for quarter-hour.

6.   Return scallops to skillet and stir to coat.

7.   Serve and enjoy!

Nutrition (Per Serving)

Calories: 417

Fat: 31g

Net Carbohydrates: 5g

Protein: 29g

Salmon and Cucumber Platter

Serving: 4

Prep Time: 10 minutes

Cook Time: nil

Ingredients:

2 cucumbers, cubed

2 teaspoons fresh squeezed lemon juice ounces non-fat yogurt teaspoon lemon zest, grated

Pepper to taste

teaspoons dill, chopped

8 ounces smoked salmon, flaked

How To:

1. Take a bowl and add cucumbers, juice, lemon peel, pepper, dill, salmon, yogurt and toss well.

2.   Serve cold.

3.   Enjoy!

Nutrition (Per Serving)

Calories: 242

Fat: 3g

Carbohydrates: 3g

Protein: 3g

Tuna Paté

Serving: 4

Prep Time: 10 minutes

Cook Time: nil

Ingredients:

ounces canned tuna, drained and flaked teaspoons fresh lemon juice 1 teaspoon onion, minced

ounces low-fat cream cheese

¼ cup parsley, chopped

How To:

1.   Take a bowl and blend in tuna, cheese, juice, parsley, onion and stir well.

2.   Serve cold and enjoy!

Nutrition (Per Serving)

Calories: 172

Fat: 2g

Carbohydrates: 8g

Protein: 4g

Beef with Pea Pods

Prep time: 5 minutes

Cook time: 10 minutes

Servings: 4

Ingredients

Thin beef steak – ¾ pound, sliced into thin strips

Peanut oil – 1 Tbsp.

Scallions – 3, sliced

Garlic – 2 cloves, minced

Minced fresh ginger – 2 tsp.

Fresh pea pods – 4 cups, trimmed

Homemade soy sauce – 3 Tbsp.

Cooked brown rice – 4 cups

Method

1. Heat the oil in a pan.

2. Add the garlic, scallions, and ginger.

3.   Stir-fry for 30 seconds.

4.   Add the sliced beef and stir-fry for 5 minutes, or until beef has browned.

5.   Add pea pods and soy sauce and stir-fry for 3 minutes.

6.   Remove from heat.

7.   Serve with rice.

Homemade soy sauce

Molasses – ¼ cup

Unflavored rice wine vinegar – 3 Tbsp.

Water – 1 Tbsp.

Sodium-free beef bouillon granules – 1 tsp.

Freshly ground black pepper - ½ tsp.

Method

1.   Mix everything in a saucepan and heat on low for 1 minute.

2.   Serve.

Nutritional Facts Per Serving

Calories: 466

Fat: 11g

Carb: 64g

Protein: 27g

Sodium 71mg

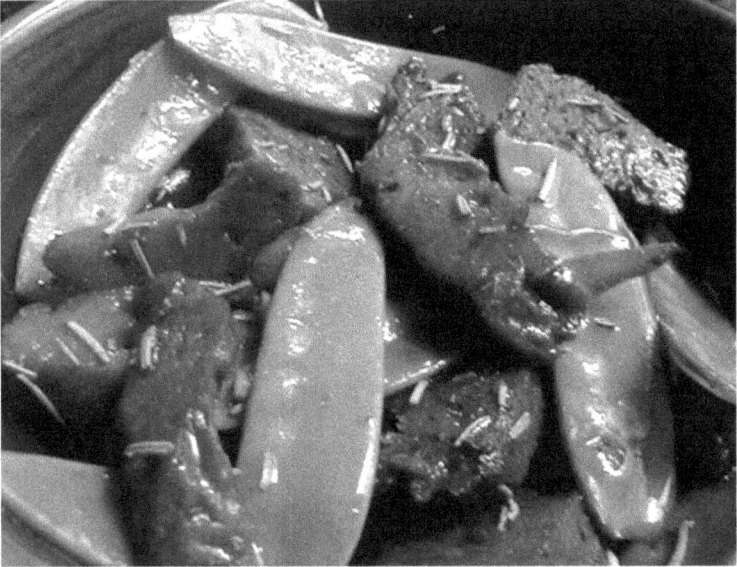

Whole-Grain Rotini with Ground Pork

Prep time: 10 minutes

Cook time: 25 minutes

Servings: 6

Ingredients

Whole-grain rotini - 1 (13-ounce) package

Lean ground pork – 1 pound

Red onion – 1, chopped

Garlic – 3 cloves, minced

Bell pepper – 1, chopped

Pumpkin puree – 1 cup Ground sage – 2 tsp.

Ground rosemary – 1 tsp.

Ground black pepper to taste

Method

1.   Cook the pasta (follow the package insturctions). Omit salt, drain and set aside.

2.   Heat a pan over medium heat. Add onion, garlic, and ground pork and sauté for 2 minutes.

3.   Add bell pepper and sauté for 5 minutes.

4.   Remove from heat. Add pasta to the pan along with remaining ingredients.

5.   Mix and serve.

Nutritional Facts Per Serving

Calories: 331

Fat: 7g

Carb: 45g

Protein: 23g

Sodium 48mg

Roasted Pork Loin with Herbs

Prep time: 20 minutes

Cook time: 1 hour

Servings: 4

Ingredients

Boneless pork loin roast – 2 lbs.

Garlic – 3 cloves, minced Dried rosemary – 1 Tbsp.

Dried thyme – 1 tsp.

Dried basil – 1 tsp.

Salt – ¼ tsp.

Olive oil – ¼ cup

White wine – ½ cup Pepper to taste

Method

1.   Preheat the oven to 350F.

2.   Crush the garlic with thyme, rosemary, basil, salt, and pepper, making a paste. Set aside.

3.   Use a knife to pierce meat several times.

4.   Press the garlic paste into the slits.

5.   Rub the meat with the rest of the garlic mixture and olive oil.

6.   Place pork loin into the oven, turning and basting with pan liquids, until the pork reaches 145F, about 1 hour. Remove the pork from the oven.

7.   Place the pan over heat and add white wine, stirring the brown bits on the bottom.

8.   Top roast with sauce.

9.   Serve.

Nutritional Facts Per Serving

Calories: 464

Fat: 20.7g

Carb: 2.4g

Protein: 59.6g

Sodium 279mg

Garlic Lime Pork Chops

Prep time: 20 minutes

Cook time: 10 minutes

Servings: 4

Ingredients

Lean boneless pork chops – 4 (6-oz. each)

Garlic – 4 cloves, crushed Cumin – ½ tsp.

Chili powder - ½ tsp.

Paprika - ½ tsp.

Juice of ½ lime Lime zest – 1 tsp.

Kosher salt - ¼ tsp.

Fresh pepper to taste

Method

1.   In a bowl, season pork with cumin, chili powder, paprika, garlic salt, and pepper. Add lime juice and zest.

2.   Marinate the pork for 20 minutes.

3.   Line a broiler pan with foil.

4.   Place the pork chops on the broiler pan and broil for 5 minutes on each side or until browned.

5.   Serve.

Nutritional Facts Per Serving

Calories: 233

Fat: 13.2g

Carb: 4.3g

Protein: 25.5g

Sodium 592mg

The Most Elegant Parsley Soufflé Ever

Serving: 5

Prep Time: 5 minutes

Cook Time: 6 minutes

Ingredients:

2 whole eggs

1 fresh red chili pepper, chopped

2 tablespoons coconut cream

1 tablespoon fresh parsley, chopped Sunflower seeds to taste

How To:

1. Pre-heat your oven to 390 degrees F.

2.   Almond butter 2 soufflé dishes.

3.   Add the ingredients to a blender and mix well.

4.   Divide batter into soufflé dishes and bake for 6 minutes.

5.   Serve and enjoy!

Nutrition (Per Serving)

Calories: 108

Fat: 9g

Carbohydrates: 9g

Protein: 6g

Fennel and Almond Bites

Serving: 12

Prep Time: 10 minutes

Cooking Time: None

Freeze Time: 3 hours

Ingredients:

1 teaspoon vanilla extract

¼ cup almond milk

¼ cup cocoa powder

½ cup almond oil

A pinch of sunflower seeds

1 teaspoon fennel seeds

How To:

1.	Take a bowl and mix the almond oil and almond milk.

2.	Beat until smooth and glossy using electric beater.

3.	Mix in the rest of the ingredients.

4.	Take a piping bag and pour into a parchment paper lined baking sheet.

5.	Freeze for 3 hours and store in the fridge.

Nutrition (Per Serving)

Total Carbs: 1g

Fiber: 1g

Protein: 1g

Fat: 20g

Feisty Coconut Fudge

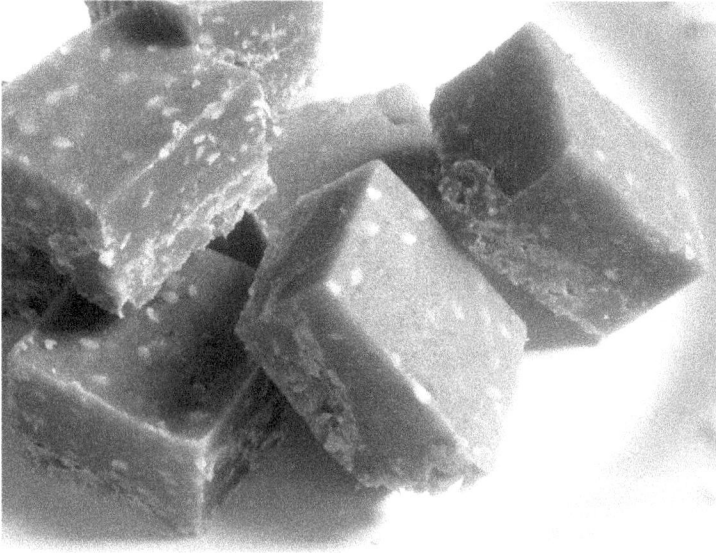

Serving: 12

Prep Time: 20 minutes

Cooking Time: None

Freeze Time: 2 hours

Ingredients:

¼ cup coconut, shredded

2 cups coconut oil

½ cup coconut cream

¼ cup almonds, chopped

1 teaspoon almond extract

A pinch of sunflower seeds

Stevia to taste

How To:

1.   Take a large bowl and pour coconut cream and coconut oil into it.

2.   Whisk using an electric beater.

3.   Whisk until the mixture becomes smooth and glossy.

4.   Add cocoa powder slowly and mix well.

5.   Add in the rest of the ingredients.

6.   Pour into a bread pan lined with parchment paper.

7.   Freeze until set.

8.   Cut them into squares and serve.

Nutrition (Per Serving)

Total Carbs: 1g

Fiber: 1g

Protein: 0g

Fat: 20g

No Bake Cheesecake

Serving: 10

Prep Time: 120 minutes

Cook Time: Nil

Ingredients:

For Crust

2 tablespoons ground flaxseeds

2 tablespoons desiccated coconut

1 teaspoon cinnamon

For Filling

4 ounces vegan cream cheese

1 cup cashews, soaked

½ cup frozen blueberries

2 tablespoons coconut oil

1 tablespoon lemon juice

1 teaspoon vanilla extract Liquid stevia

How To:

1.   Take a container and mix in the crust ingredients, mix well.

2.   Flatten the mixture at the bottom to prepare the crust of your cheesecake.

3.   Take a blender/ food processor and add the filling ingredients, blend until smooth.

4.   Gently pour the batter on top of your crust and chill for 2 hours.

5.   Serve and enjoy!

Nutrition (Per Serving)

Calories: 182

Fat: 16g

Carbohydrates: 4g

Protein: 3g

Easy Chia Seed Pumpkin Pudding

Serving: 4

Prep Time: 10-15 minutes/ overnight chill time

Cook Time: Nil

Ingredients:

1 cup maple syrup

2 teaspoons pumpkin spice

1 cup pumpkin puree

1 ¼ cup almond milk

½ cup chia seeds

How To:

1.   Add all of the ingredients to a bowl and gently stir.

2.   Let it refrigerate overnight or at least 15 minutes.

3.   Top with your desired ingredients, such as blueberries, almonds, etc.

4.   Serve and enjoy!

Nutrition (Per Serving)

Calories: 230

Fat: 10g

Carbohydrates:22g

Protein:11g

Lovely Blueberry Pudding

Serving: 4

Prep Time: 20 minutes

Cook Time: Nil

Ingredients:

2 cups frozen blueberries

2 teaspoons lime zest, grated freshly

20 drops liquid stevia

2 small avocados, peeled, pitted and chopped ½ teaspoon fresh ginger, grated freshly

4 tablespoons fresh lime juice

10 tablespoons water

How To:

1.   Add all of the listed ingredients to a blender (except blueberries) and pulse the mixture well.

2.   Transfer the mix into small serving bowls and chill the bowls.

3.   Serve with a topping of blueberries.

4.   Enjoy!

Nutrition (Per Serving)

Calories: 166

Fat: 13g

Carbohydrates: 13g

Protein: 1.7g

Decisive Lime and Strawberry Popsicle

Serving: 4

Prep Time: 2 hours

Cook Time: Nil

Ingredients:

1 tablespoon lime juice, fresh

¼ cup strawberries, hulled and sliced

¼ cup coconut almond milk, unsweetened and full fat 2
teaspoons natural sweetener

How To:

1.   Blend the listed ingredients in a blender until smooth.

2.   Pour mix into popsicle molds and let them chill for 2
hours.

3.   Serve and enjoy!

Nutrition (Per Serving)

Calories: 166

Fat: 17g

Carbohydrates: 3g

Protein: 1g

Authentic Ginger and Berry Smoothie

Serving: 2

Prep Time: 5 minutes

Cook Time: Nil

Ingredients:

2 cups blackberries

2 cups unsweetened almond milk

1 -2 packs of stevia

1 piece of 1-inch fresh ginger, peeled and roughly chopped

2 cups crushed ice

How To:

1.   Add the listed ingredients to a blender and blend the whole mixture until smooth.

2.   Serve chilled and enjoy!

Nutrition (Per Serving)

Calories: 200

Fat: 10g

Carbohydrates: 14g

Protein 2g

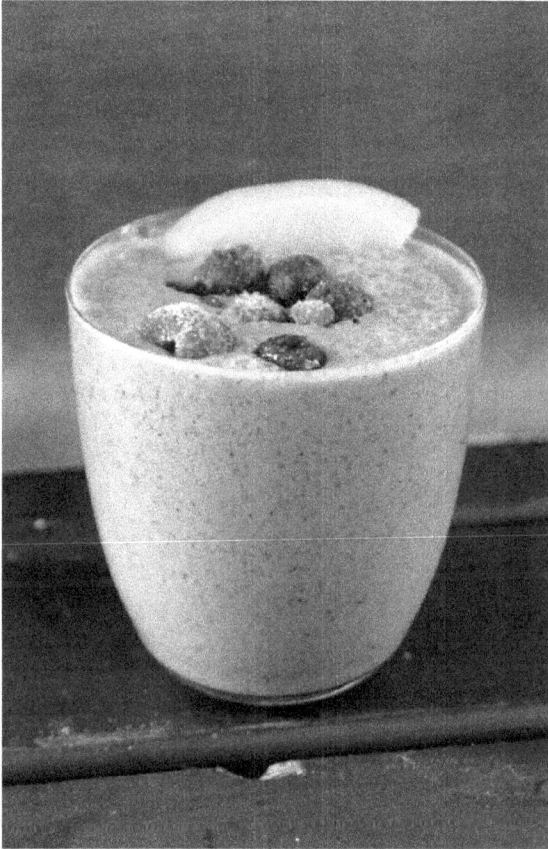

A Glassful of Kale and Spinach

Serving: 2

Prep Time: 5 minutes

Ingredients:

Handful of kale

Handful of spinach

2 broccoli heads

1 tomato

Handful of lettuce

1 avocado, cubed

1 cucumber, cubed

Juice of ½ lemon

Pineapple juice as needed

How To:

1.   Add all the listed ingredients to your blender.

2.   Blend until smooth.

3. Add a few ice cubes and serve the smoothie.

4. Enjoy!

Nutrition (Per Serving)

Calories: 200

Fat: 10g

Carbohydrates: 14g

Protein 2g

Green Tea, Turmeric, and Mango Smoothie

Serving: 2

Prep Time: 5 minutes

Ingredients:

2 cups mango, cubed

2 teaspoons turmeric powder

2 tablespoons Green Tea powder

2 cups almond milk

2 tablespoons honey

1 cup crushed ice

How To:

1.   Add the listed ingredients to a blender and blend the whole mixture until smooth.

2.   Serve chilled and enjoy!

Nutrition (Per Serving)

Calories: 200

Fat: 10g

Carbohydrates: 14g

Protein 2g

The Great Anti-Oxidant Glass

Serving: 2

Prep Time: 5 minutes

Ingredients:

1 whole ripe avocado

4 cups organic baby spinach leaves

1 cup filtered water

Juice of 1 lemon

1 English cucumber, chopped

3 stems fresh parsley

5 stems fresh mint

1-inch piece fresh ginger

2 large ice cubes

How To:

1.   Add all the listed ingredients to your blender.

2.   Blend until smooth.

3.   Add a few ice cubes and serve the smoothie.

4.   Enjoy!

Nutrition (Per Serving)

Calories: 200

Fat: 10g

Carbohydrates: 14g

Protein 2g

Fresh Minty Smoothie

Serving: 1

Prep Time: 10 minutes

Ingredients:

1 stalk celery

2 cups water

2 ounces almonds

1 packet stevia

1 cup spinach

2 mint leaves

How To:

1. Add listed ingredients to blender.

2. Blend until you have a smooth and creamy texture.

3. Serve chilled and enjoy!

Nutrition (Per Serving)

Calories: 417

Fat: 43g

Carbohydrates: 10g

Protein: 5.5g

Apple Slices

Serving: 4

Prep Time: 10 minutes

Cook Time: 10 minutes

Ingredients:

1 cup of coconut oil

¼ cup date paste

2 tablespoons ground cinnamon

4 granny smith apples, peeled and sliced, cored

How To:

1.   Take a large sized skillet and place it over medium heat.

2.   Add oil and allow the oil to heat up.

3.   Stir in cinnamon and date paste into the oil.

4.   Add cut up apples and cook for 5-8 minutes until crispy.

5.   Serve and enjoy!

Nutrition (Per Serving)

Calories: 368

Fat: 23g

Carbohydrates: 44g

Protein: 1g

Elegant Cashew Sauce

Serving: 4

Prep Time: 5 minutes

Cook Time: Nil

Ingredients:

3 ounces cashew nuts

¼ cup water

½ cup olive oil

1 tablespoons lemon juice

½ teaspoon onion powder

½ teaspoon sunflower seeds

1 pinch cayenne pepper

How To:

Add nuts to your blender and process.

Add other ingredients (except oil) and process until smooth.

Add a little bit of oil and puree.

Serve as needed!

Nutrition (Per Serving)

Calories: 361

Fat: 37g

Carbohydrates: 6g

Protein: 3g

Lovely Japanese Cabbage Dish

Serving: 6

Prep Time: 25 minutes

Cook Time: Nil

Ingredients:

3 tablespoons sesame oil

3 tablespoons rice vinegar

1 garlic clove, minced

1 teaspoon fresh ginger root, grated

1 teaspoon sunflower seeds

1 teaspoon pepper

½ large head cabbage, cored and shredded 1 bunch green onions, thinly sliced 1 cup almond slivers

¼ cup toasted sesame seeds

How To:

1.   Add all listed ingredients to a large bowl, making sure to add the wet ingredients first, followed by the dried ingredients.

2.   Toss well to ensure that the cabbages are coated well.

3.   Let it chill and enjoy!

Nutrition (Per Serving)

Calories: 126

Fat: 10g

Carbohydrates: 9g

Protein: 4g

Almond Buttery Green Cabbage

Serving: 4

Prep Time: 10 minutes

Cook Time: 15 minutes

Ingredients:

1 ½ pounds shredded green cabbage

3 ounces almond butter

Sunflower seeds and pepper to taste

1 dollop, whipped cream

How To:

1.   Take a large skillet and place it over medium heat.

2.   Add almond butter and melt.

3.   Stir in cabbage and sauté for 15 minutes.

4.   Season accordingly.

5.   Serve with a dollop of cream.

6.   Enjoy!

Nutrition (Per Serving)

Calories: 199

Fat: 17g

Carbohydrates: 10g

Protein: 3g

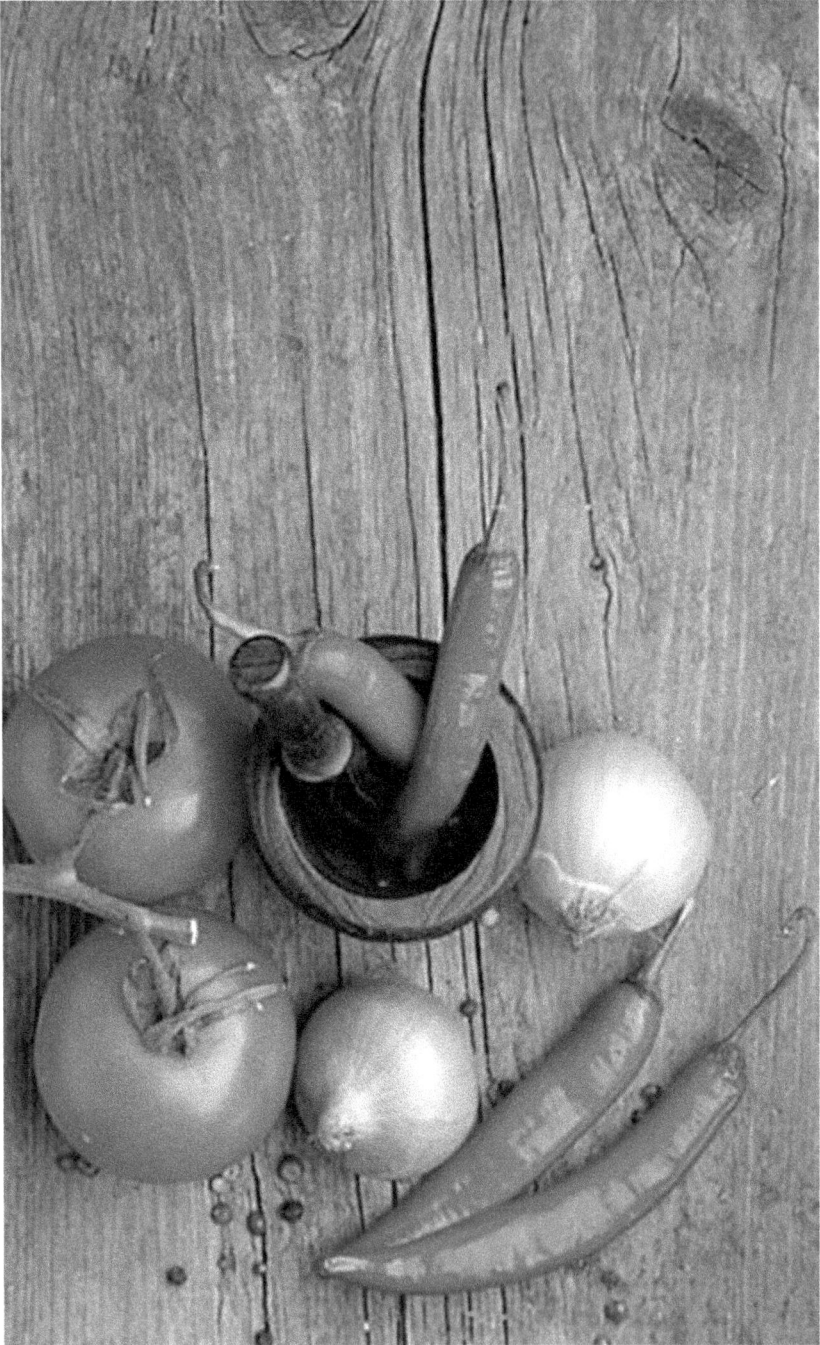

www.ingramcontent.com/pod-product-compliance
Lightning Source LLC
Chambersburg PA
CBHW071109030426
42336CB00013BA/2016